Kendra

Kendra

A Story of God's Providence

Bobbi Aker Campbell

The Wooster Book Company
Wooster • Ohio

The Wooster Book Company
205 West Liberty Street • Wooster Ohio • 44691

Published in the United States of America.

ISBN 1-888683-16-3

Library of Congress Cataloging-In-Publication Data

Campbell, Bobbi Aker, 1946 –
Kendra : a story of God's providence / Bobbi Aker Campbell.
p. cm.
Includes bibliographical references.
ISBN 1-888683-16-3 (alk. paper)
1. Shultzman, Kendra. 2. Food allergy—Patients—United States—Religious life. 3. Asthmatics—United States—Religious life. 4. Christian biography—United States I. Title

BR1725.S4658C36 1997
248.8'61'092—dc21
[B] 97-21603
CIP
AC

This book is printed on acid-free paper.

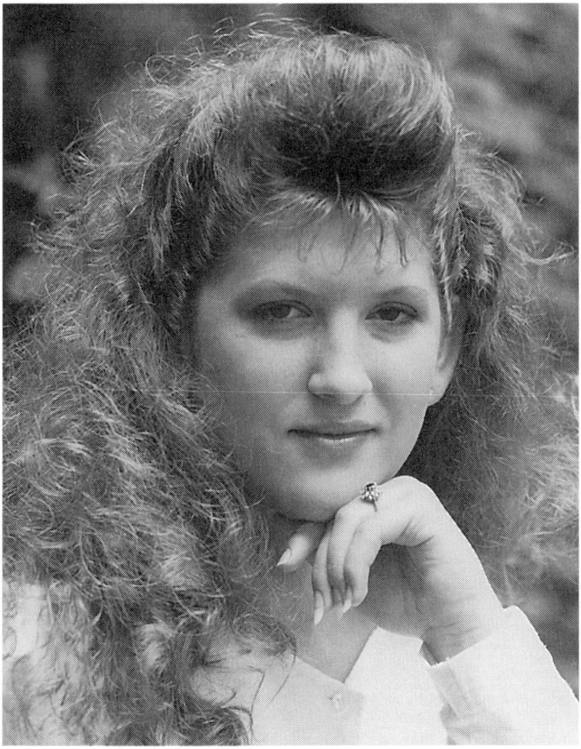

To Kendra –

Who lived life fully growing up,

and lives Life fully now.

Teach us to number our days aright,
that we may gain a heart of wisdom.

—Psalms 90:12

Kendra

Chapter One

THE OLD MERCEDES TRUCK bounced and slid on the mud rutted road. The temperature was climbing to 110 degrees outside the open window. The African savanna spread out to the horizon. Terry, Bonnie, Kendra, and Aaron Shultzman were heading to Baoro, Central African Republic, on a missionary trip. The roads were barely passable at the end of the rainy season, and the bridges were weakened.

The Shultzmans started across a bridge and saw that part of the timber roadbed had collapsed. Terry found some local villagers to help him drag over a log to fill in the hole. The choice was to repair the bridge, or make a one hundred mile detour. Declaring it now *safe*, Terry drove the truck over the bridge and continued their trip. The next bridge appeared intact and the Shultzman's proceeded across it. Suddenly the old Mercedes truck lurched to the right. Bonnie found herself staring out to the river below the window. The embankment had given way and the front tire was hanging over the edge. Terry built a support pile of stones under the tire and the family continued on their way. They were going to have enough adventure experiences to last a lifetime.

Terry and Bonnie had met in Ohio and married while attending Grace College in Indiana. Terry became a skilled brick-layer to help pay his college expenses. After college, they moved to Colorado Springs. The area was growing rapidly and masonry workers were in demand. Terry and Bonnie explored the mountains on the weekends. Their car tires often slid on the gravelly scree and safety seemed tenuous, but they met the challenge of driving on the narrow, rimless mountain roads.

The first months in Colorado were exciting for them. They were exploring a new part of the country and their first child was born a few months after their move. Kendra's birth opened up the beginning of family life for them. Bonnie cherished her daughter and Terry was overwhelmed by his loving response to Kendra. They continued their weekend jaunts and included Kendra in their travels to the upper mountain regions and trails that they had discovered.

The Shultzmans heard of a need for workers to help Missions Aviation Fellowship with a building project in Bogata, Columbia. The idea of using their skills to help others was exciting. They found that their interest in foreign mission service grew. They began to explore the idea of going to South America, but then later selected an opportunity for service in Africa through the Grace Brethren Church. They saw the need in the Central African Republic for Terry's building skills and Bonnie's teaching degree.

The decision to go so far away was not easy, but Terry and Bonnie felt that God was calling them and would provide protection wherever it was needed. Kendra's toddler years were spent in Quebec and Switzerland as her parents enrolled in French language study courses.

Kendra was almost three when the Shultzmans finally arrived at Bata in the Central African Republic. The missionary compound was a big playground for Kendra. She rode her tricycle sent by Grandma and Grandpa in America. She loved the goats that wandered the compound area and the lizards that climbed the walls. She learned the native trade language, *Sango*, even before her parents did. Kendra needed *Sango* to play with the village children!

Linda Kay lived in the compound and became Kendra's first friend. The two girls played with their dolls as they sat in the African dirt. Kendra had another companion after her brother Aaron was born. Her closest friends were Heidi and Stephanie. They became Kendra's "sisters." They lived at a different mission station, but during visits the three girls were so inseparable that they gained the name of "The Three Musketeers."

The Shultzman's home at the Bata compound combined American furniture and African reality. Generators produced electricity during part of each day, gas ran the refrigerator, and laundry was an all day occupation. Bonnie and Terry adjusted to the local culture and learned the native language. Terry spent his time repairing buildings in the mission's compound and constructing new buildings. Bonnie assumed responsibility for teaching at some Bible Institute classes.

The extended missionary family helped the Shultzmans in their adjustment to Africa. These more experienced missionaries understood the stress of learning to live and speak in a foreign culture. The Shultzmans, however, had an additional and more serious adjustment to make—Kendra was severely allergic to many foods and constant vigilance was necessary to protect her health.

While still in Colorado, Bonnie and Terry had stopped to eat dinner on the way to the grocery store. Kendra was six months old and was being breast fed. At the restaurant, they gave Kendra a small sip of milk to hold her hunger until they got home. Kendra dozed off and then awakened suddenly with projectile vomiting. Afterwards, she remained groggy and slept all evening.

The next day was her six-month-old check-up. The doctor felt that Kendra had a reaction to the sip of milk at the restaurant. This was the beginning of the Shultzmans' growing discoveries of the range of foods which caused Kendra difficulty. Over the next two years, Bonnie learned to read labels carefully and keep dairy products away from Kendra.

On the very night that they arrived in Africa, they had the joy of greeting their extended missionary family and the dismay of needing to seek emergency care for the first time for Kendra.

The Shultzmans were welcomed at Banqui with a gathering at a potluck supper. It had been a long day for them flying from Switzerland. The warmth of the fellowship was a real delight. The main dish was a "Johnny Marzetti" casserole with cheese on top. Bonnie carefully removed the cheese and gave Kendra some of the noodles below. About an hour later, Kendra broke out with huge hives on her scalp and began screaming from abdominal pain. Even though the top layer of the casserole had been removed, the oil from the cheese had passed down into the noodles and triggered the hives and severe abdominal distress. The Shultzmans rushed Kendra to the local hospital and were thankful that adequate emergency care was available. Kendra received medication which gave her relief.

Kendra was too young to understand the seriousness of her food allergies. Bonnie struggled to find those foods which were safe for her daughter and to keep her away from those which caused problems. Kendra had a gentle, compliant personality and if her folks said that she wasn't to eat a certain food, she stayed away from it. However, even with the Shultzmans' vigilance, and Kendra's compliance, it was difficult to avoid allergic reactions.

The main staple food was peanuts, bought from farmers who sold their crop door to door. Peanuts were a safe food for Kendra as long as they were cooked. A neighbor let Kendra chew on some peanuts for a snack, and the raw peanuts gave Kendra an allergic reaction.

Another day, Kendra sat at a neighbor's table and ate some potato chips. Within an hour, she had an allergy attack. Bonnie and her friend found out that a piece of cheese had laid on that part of the table earlier. Once again a trace of oil from the cheese was the culprit.

The vigilance to protect Kendra was constant and wearing. Terry and Bonnie knew that even though the other missionaries loved Kendra, they could not understand the strain endured trying to watch over her food. A favorite missionary "aunt" asked Bonnie if Kendra could have a piece of cake. Bonnie reviewed the list of ingredients with her friend and agreed that all seemed okay. Kendra enjoyed her treat and licked her lips. An hour later she became violently ill and was covered with hives. Dr. Walker, a missionary physician friend visiting in the home, was able to give an antihistamine shot which stabilized Kendra. The Shultzmans were grateful that again medical care was available when Kendra needed it quickly.

But Bonnie still lived with the guilty feeling of failing to protect her daughter. What had happened? The hostess recalled that in making the treat this particular time, she had substituted the regular ingredient of BLUE BAND MARGARINE with some left over pieces of baking chocolate. The margarine was a safe food for Kendra, but the trace of butter in the chocolate set off the reaction.

Terry shared the sense of guilt at not always being able to protect his daughter. Sunday brunch was one of the highlights of the week. It was a time to relax with other missionaries. One Sunday, Terry enjoyed conversation and laughter with a friend over the brunch table. Terry held Kendra on his knee, and talked with his friend of the difficulties Bonnie and he had protecting Kendra from her food allergies. "If she even touches the food she is allergic to, she gets a reaction."

The friend listened sympathetically. He knew how this allergy stress was adding to the Shultzman's adjustment of living in a foreign culture. He finished his coffee, gave Kendra a good-bye peck on her cheek, and left. A few minutes later, Terry sat at the same table holding Kendra and comforting her as her face broke out in hives. The friend had put cream in his coffee. His good-bye peck contained a trace of dairy product that was too much for Kendra.

Terry also experienced some of Bonnie's frustration in trying to provide safe foods which Kendra could eat. Bonnie went away for a few days and

Kendra's allergies were acute. The whole time Bonnie was gone, all that Terry could find to safely feed Kendra was hamburger and potatoes. That's all Kendra ate for three meals each day. She never complained.

Kendra had some allergy tests run when she was four years old. Patches of selected potential allergens were placed across her back. The whole test sequence had to be repeated. Kendra's reaction to the allergens was so strong that the patch areas blurred into one another, and the doctor could not determine which allergens were the culprit.

Dr. Mason, a missionary friend, visited Bonnie and Terry. He told them that as parents Kendra was in their trust. No one else was going to be as vigilant as they in watching out for her. The Shultzmans began to tote picnics for Kendra whenever they were invited over to other homes. Bonnie began to send safe snacks with Kendra when she was invited to play. The only way to really protect Kendra was to be the only providers of her food.

After four years in Africa, the Shultzmans moved briefly to California and then back to their home state of Ohio. As they readjusted to the American culture, they continued in their effort to be the only providers of food for Kendra. At each school where they enrolled Kendra, the Shultzmans went to the principal and explained the importance of Kendra *not* receiving any treats or eating any birthday cake served at class parties. One principal indicated clearly that he thought they were over-protective parents.

In addition, just after their return, Kendra's physician heard the wheezing of asthma when he examined Kendra. She would now have to watch her activity level as well as her food.

Kendra seemed unaffected by all of the attention to her health. She included information on her allergies as part of her "introduction" to her new class. Years later, a classmate's mother wrote, "I remember Lisa coming home in second or third grade announcing, 'We have a new girl, her name is Kendra and she has lots of allergies so she brings her lunch. She's really nice!'"*

Kendra's compliant nature was housed in a tender heart. During her second grade year, she wrote a "letter to Mommy" in church:

> I Love Mommy
> and Daddy and
> aaron. God is the first
> one on the List—maybe
> not on others But on
> mine he is so Loving
> and kind and good and
> sweet it's Because
> he Loves us. and we
> Love him. and he mite
> be Aarons Christ too

I wrot this litter
Because I've been keeping
this inside my heart
Love Kendra*

Kendra was well liked in elementary school. She had a great sense of humor and the ability to entertain as a story-teller. She amused others with her anecdotes of everyday life. One time, there was a canoeing mishap with girls from her church. Kendra comically recounted sitting in the water after the canoe capsized and watching the soggy sandwiches from their picnic lunch bags float down the river.

Kendra also showed a flair for writing. Each spring, her school participated in a Young Authors program. Two children from each class were invited to attend the conference. Kendra was selected three years in a row. In the sixth grade, Kendra asked her mom if it was okay if she didn't write a book that year so that other children would have a chance to be selected. Kendra looked for ways to put others first and to encourage them.

Sometimes the trips out of town to the allergy specialist's office would become social events for Kendra and her mom. They would each take a friend and make a day of it. Saralyn, a friend from church and school, remembered going with Kendra to Columbus for an appointment and then spending the day shopping. Though Kendra handled her allergies without complaint, Saralyn recalled that Kendra tried to limit her discomfort. At one visit Kendra begged the doctor to do her allergy testing on her arm rather than all over her back. "I won't scratch at them. I promise," she told him.

Kendra continued to be compliant in avoiding the foods that could harm her and was trustworthy in approaching her parents quickly for medication if she sensed a reaction developing. Kendra did not like taking medicine. When she asked for medicine, her parents knew that she needed it.

The Shultzmans kept their home available as the center of Kendra's social life with friends. Most sleepovers were at Kendra's home. The other girls enjoyed the laughing and story telling of Terry and Bonnie, who at the same time were able to make sure that Kendra got only safe food and drinks. Kendra's girl friends never thought much about her allergies but knew that when you went to Kendra's house, you washed your hands after eating. The hand washing was important so that nothing on their hands would rub off on something that Kendra would later touch.

Kendra's need to take medication for asthma and to avoid many foods became part of her everyday life at school. As her classmates became increasingly active in sports and rougher playground activities, Kendra had to limit the extent of her exercise. The asthma was affected by heat or cold which sometimes caused hives and wheezing. She also had many inhalant allergies like dust, mold and pollen. Her food allergies could also cause a wheezing asthmatic reaction. Yet Kendra's humor and acceptance of her limitations helped her friends feel comfortable around her.

One time at school, Kendra needed her asthma medication. Her friend Aleta accompanied her down to the principal's office where her inhaler was kept. Aleta told a joke just at the wrong moment, and Kendra snorted as she laughed. They both howled as they realized that the medication was then coming out of Kendra's nose. Kendra's willingness to laugh at herself helped others accept her and not be overly concerned about her asthma and allergies. Kendra depended on her friends to help her achieve that sense of being "normal." Her friendships were based on what the friends had in common, rather than their differences.

It was the move to Wooster that caused Kendra to realize how important friendships were for her sense of acceptance and normalcy. Kendra later wrote:

> *From the time I was born, my family had always moved around; six months in one state, a year in another. For four years we even moved out of the country. …*
>
> *Once I started school, my parents realized the importance of staying in one place. My dad found a job in a quaint little town in southern Ohio. My*

> *friendships no longer consisted of only* can Susie come out and play? *I had now graduated to sleep-overs. My first real friendships were beginning to develop. I realized the importance of choosing good friends that really cared.*
>
> *Then one day the announcement came that we were moving again. I was very upset and angry with my parents. How could they do this to me? …*
>
> *On my very last day in Caldwell, everyone treated me with every kindness imaginable…*
>
> *I will always remember this day because I learned the value of friendship. I learned that in the hardest times, special friends that care always make things easier. I learned that friendship is what makes life worthwhile.**

As Kendra grew towards adolescence, her friendships at school became even more critical. She began to face the peer pressure of young teens. Being different became reason enough to exclude a classmate from the group.

Chapter Two

WHEN KENDRA BEGAN ATTENDING Triway Junior High School, she drew the curious attention of new classmates who asked, "Why aren't you having the pizza?" and "Why do you always bring your lunch?" and "Why do you take all of those medicines?" etc. In addition, some of her elementary classmates now found her allergies and asthma fair game for teasing. "Put downs" are the way junior high students handle their own insecurities by pointing out classmates' weaknesses.

Kendra used her acceptance of herself and her gift of laughter to help others feel comfortable around her and to keep herself in the social flow at school. She chose to answer her new classmates' curious questions without embarrassment and to laugh along with her former classmates without taking offense. In making these choices, Kendra avoided letting her health differences isolate her from the crowd.

But Kendra knew that her food restrictions and asthma did set her apart. She remained fragile on the inside to the food and activity limitations that made her different. Though she didn't show any outward embarrassment or hurt, she inwardly yearned to be seen as totally normal.

Her close group of friends gave Kendra the sense of "normal" that she sought. Five or six friends continued to have over-nights at the Shultzmans throughout the junior high years The girls would freeze on the back porch trying to stay awake to see the sun rise and then come inside and practice aerobics at 6 A.M. Kendra's great sense of humor and her laugh were contagious. Her funny comments and observations kept the group laughing.

Laurie became Kendra's best friend during junior high. The girls lived in different school districts but knew each other through church. Each Sunday afternoon they met at youth group and spent time together.

The two discussed the important issues of their life as young teenagers. The first area was make-up and trying to look older. They schemed over how to purchase and wear more make-up than they were allowed, and how to do it without their parents noticing. They discussed their "boy friends." They helped each other figure out who liked them or helped gather information on boys they liked.

Kendra gained increased independence in her social life during these youth group afternoons and increased independence in eating away from home. The Shultzmans explored ways to allow Kendra more freedom to eat with her friends. Surprisingly, one of the easiest places for Kendra to eat safely was at a fast food restaurant. The fast food chains were franchised and standardized in food purchase and production. The Shultzmans experimented with items on the menus and developed a list of "safe" foods for Kendra to order.

However, just as they had found in Africa, even with all of their careful planning they could not always protect Kendra from an allergic reaction. One Sunday, Kendra and Laurie walked to a fast food restaurant during a junior high youth activity. They carried their burgers back to church and ate. An hour later, Kendra called her dad and told him to come pick her up and take her to the Emergency Room. By the time Terry arrived, Kendra was getting numb. Terry told Kendra to swallow some of the medication which she always carried. Kendra responded "Dad, you don't understand! This is an emergency." It took the Emergency Room staff four hours to stabilize her condition and to be certain that she was out of danger.

What had happened? Laurie and Kendra had laughed and talked their way through their meal. Neither of them thought anything of it when Laurie offered Kendra the last bite of the hamburger which she couldn't finish, nor did either remember it was actually a cheeseburger. There was not enough cheese on the last bite for Kendra to taste beneath the ketchup and pickle, but there was enough present to set off her allergy.

This incident was the most serious allergic incident Kendra had yet experienced. She had her first anaphylactic reaction. The Shultzmans faced once again the fact that Kenra's allergies were life-threatening. Their parental instinct was to draw Kendra back in closer to home and be her only source of food, but Kendra was growing up and needed to be given the opportunity to increase her independence.

Kendra ate at school each day from a lunch bag brought from home. On weekends, she often ate out with a group of friends at the fast food places. But one of the most difficult places to balance growing independence with safe food was at the youth retreats which Kendra attended several times a year. The length of the retreats required multiple meals to be eaten in a strange camp setting.

At first, Bonnie volunteered to accompany the youth group as the resident "cook." She helped make the meal for the entire group, and would also make an alternative meal for Kendra. The group's lasagna with cheese might be paired with Kendra's plate of spaghetti without cheese. Other campers remember Bonnie coming along on the retreats and Kendra saying wistfully, "I wish my mom wasn't here." The fellow campers understood—who would want Mom coming to camp with you? But Kendra's wish never developed into a complaint in her mom's presence. Kendra understood that Bonnie also wished that the need for her presence didn't exist. Kendra was aware of her mom's concern for her safety, and she wanted to cooperate to help her mom be as worry free as possible.

Sometimes Kendra had to admit that her allergies prevented her from joining in an activity. At a junior high retreat, the group was putting together shish-kabobs to grill. Kendra backed away from the table and said, "I am allergic to that." The pineapple juice was burning her skin. Her friends understood that she couldn't participate, but they did not really understand how a food allergy could irritate from just touching and not even eating a food.

Others were helpful in trying to serve food that was acceptable for Kendra. At Bell Choir parties, the director made sure that the party food being planned could be enjoyed by Kendra. Saralyn also had some minor food allergies and recalled that it was sometimes humorous to find enough food to enjoy to which they each weren't allergic.

Even though her mom's presence indicated a severe medical condition, Kendra herself never spoke of her allergies to others outside the family. She used her mom as her confidant for fears and questions, but kept discussions with friends filled with those things which were normal in her life. By not mentioning her differences, she increased her sense of belonging by being like everyone else.

Years later, Kendra expressed her feelings:

> *… growing up, I had many problems with allergies and asthma. When I went to retreats, or things where food was prepared ahead of time, I had to bring my own food. This was embarrassing for me because everyone would always make a big deal about it and ask why I wasn't eating what was prepared, etc. It seems like kind of a foolish thing to be embarrassed about, but I was. This also caused me to want to be 'normal, just like everyone else.' These attitudes were strongly built up in my mind by the time I reached adolescence.*[*]

It was the understanding of her friends and family that helped Kendra get through the early adolescent years. It was Kendra's determination to make the best of her allergies without making them the center of attention. It was her friends' determination to allow Kendra her privacy in this area and treat any required restraints as acceptable. Life is always easier when there is someone who understands and accepts you as you are. Kendra had to adjust to losing the ready companionship of the friend who understood her best. In August before ninth grade, Laurie moved to Columbus, Ohio. Kendra wrote this farewell:

Laurie,

I want to thank you for the past few years
when you've been there to share my laughter
and you've been there to share my tears.

You've been my very best friend
And I pray we'll always be,
For only God could know
How special you are to me.

Hey! Think positive!! This isn't the end of our friendship. It's just the beginning of a new part of it. I know it'll be hard at first, but, ya know, without changes, we don't grow. Only as high as I reach can I grow. If you *ever* need someone I'll always be here for you. To talk to you, to listen to you, & to dream with you. I don't [know] what I'd do without you. But God can give us the strength to carry on. No matter where we are, what the circumstance may be. Even though I may not always be with you in person, I'll *always* be with you in my mind.

I love you.

Friends
Forever,

Kendra*

By these mid-teen years, Kendra had gained some independence from her family and was enjoying acceptance with her peers. She looked forward to high school to continue growing up and becoming more independent.

Chapter Three

THE SHULTZMANS' SENSE OF HUMOR and ability to laugh at one another made their home a respite for Kendra during her high school years. Kendra had strong relationships with each member of her family.

Kendra and Bonnie shared a close friendship. During the later high school years, Bonnie and Kendra moved cautiously through areas of disagreement as Kendra worked out her teenage need for increased freedom and personal responsibility. Kendra never complained to her friends about disagreements she had with Bonnie. Instead, she expressed her support and thanks for all her mother did for her. They spent time shopping, talking, and creating humor around the house. Terry and Aaron were often the brunt of their humor.

Terry continued to consider Kendra one of the treasures in his life. He prized their relationship and communication. Some of Kendra's friends watched with envy the loving, teasing relationship shared by

Terry and Kendra. Terry could talk with Kendra and was so pleased that Kendra also sensed his understanding of what she said to him. He was surprised when she confided her feelings of inferiority. In Terry's eyes, he saw her as vivacious and confident.

Aaron considered Kendra his best friend and she reciprocated. Kendra brought Aaron to youth group activities with her even before he was officially old enough. She teased him about any "other" girl friends he had besides her.

Bonnie and Kendra used their gift of humor to lighten their requisite conversation before Kendra went places by herself. Instead of reviewing a routine checklist for the medications Kendra needed to carry, they made up nicknames. They created an image of a social gala to accompany Kendra. Bonnie called out, "Are your friends going with you? Do you have Ben, Al, Ven and Theo?" These were their code names for her medications; Benadryl, Alupent, Ventolin and Theodur.

Kendra used Bonnie as her friend for talking about her frustrations and fears about her health. Kendra continued not to speak of these things outside of her family. She minimized her food reactions and the role asthma played in limiting her exertions. She focused no attention on her allergies or asthma in front of her friends. Sometimes, she would use her inhaler more often than prescribed because she did not want to stop her activity. She told Saralyn once, "Don't tell my

Mom." Her quiet attempt to live life just a little differently than her parents wanted was a typical adolescent choice and her friends understood it. But privately, Kendra continued to feel insecure and different.

As a teenager, babysitting offered Kendra a steady source of income. At times, her allergies compromised her ability to carry out that task. One night, she went to a family's home to babysit. After being in the house for a while, she began to react to food allergies in the moist air left over from the steamy cooking. She began to have trouble breathing. Kendra called her home. Terry brought the children back to their home, while Bonnie took Kendra to the Emergency Room.

Food reactions occurred even at home. If Bonnie made cookies with butter for the rest of the family, she needed to make sure that the baking was done when Kendra was not at home. Kendra would start wheezing if she walked into the kitchen and there was still moist air from the baking or from bubbling pots cooking on the stove.

Laurie E moved to Wooster during high school. She met Kendra in school and began attending the same church. The two girls often drove to Sunday evening youth activities together. Laurie observed how often Kendra needed to use her inhaler when they walked or spent time together. She also knew that her purse was full of medications. But, the two never discussed the extent of Kendra's allergies and asthma. Their relationship was another tribute to the friendships that Kendra maintained. She had friends who shared the joys and tribulations of being a teenager without being bothered by the limitations of her health.

Kendra also continued her friendship with her other friend Laurie in Columbus through letters and calls. In their letters, they covered topics that were hard for teenagers to voice face to face. These letters gave Kendra a private confidante with whom to share what she was thinking behind her front of "normalcy." She and Laurie questioned what it was like to be growing up and what they wanted out of life. In the midst of adolescence, neither girl could imagine being older than twenty.

Kendra's closest friends were from her youth group, but they were in the minority in high school where many students were not active in church related activities. Acceptance in the larger high school group was based on common teenage social norms including wearing the right clothes, acting cool, and, if necessary, making fun at the expense of others. Kendra and her friends were proud to be included in a larger group at school. However, there were also times in high school when her private world of faith and the pressure of her peer group collided.

Kendra quietly expressed her faith in classes when the discussion was relevant. She mentioned her involvement in her youth group. Kendra and Saralyn were in the same speech class one year. They divided up details about the summer youth conference so that between their two introductory speeches, the class would have a good overview of all that the girls had learned at the conference. The two girls were also in French class together, and during the year, they each had a chance to quietly share about their Christian faith.

Sometimes class interactions did not go so smoothly. Once, during her senior year, Kendra was sitting in English class with a group of friends. They were having a great time laughing and enjoying one another's company. The teacher handed out a story to finish with several proposed beginnings. One of the group, who was also in youth group with Kendra, glanced over the paragraphs and then spoke out, "I think that this is about Satan." The entire class laughed, including Kendra. Later, Kendra regretted that she had not been more supportive of a spiritual concern. Kendra's embarrassment showed the tension that she felt between joining in with the group reaction versus supporting a friend whose expression of faith was ridiculed.

Kendra later used her writing skills to express her ambivalent feelings from this time in school:

> *My adolescence was a time of serious self-identity crisis, a great time of internal struggle.*

> *The struggle...was the struggle between wanting to be accepted by my peers, wanting to be like everyone else, and wanting to live a life that would be pleasing to God. In my high school, I knew few Christians. Most of my friends were friends only to a point because I didn't live for the same things that they did. I felt uncomfortable going to parties with them because of the immense pressure to do exactly the opposite of what God would want me to do.*
>
> *There were many times though, that I wanted to forget about God. I wanted to have friends that I would be able to understand, and that would be able to understand and accept me. Many times I was frustrated because I didn't want to just have Christian friends. I did not want to run and hide from the world because they were different than me, but at the same time, I desperately needed friends that I could relate to. I was very tired of the game of compromising just enough to fit in, but not enough to actually "stray from God." I was also tired of not being either one way or the other—not being free from my conscience enough to be able to fit in with my friends, and not living life with the power of God.**

Kendra chose not to walk away from this spiritual struggle but to work it through. It was the same attitude that had helped her keep a good outward attitude about her allergies and asthma and to not live with self-pity. Youth group at church and youth conferences helped focus her attention on spiritual issues.

At one retreat, the group created the *World's Biggest Milkshake.* They lined a garbage can, threw in milk, ice cream, syrup, and used a huge electric drill to stir it up. The crowd laughed hilariously as the milkshake sprayed its way across the room. While the rest of the crowd grabbed at the spray, Kendra watched from the other side of the kitchen. Dan Travis, her youth pastor, had cautioned her ahead of time that the activity might be dangerous for her. She was able to join in the general fun but was not free to abandon herself to the activity. A drop of the spraying cream might land on her skin and cause a reaction. She needed to control her exposure to the risk involved.

Pastor Dan reflected, "[There is] no doubt in my mind that she understood that this was a matter of life and death. She had been close to death a couple of times. I think that has an impact—probably more than the average kid. It really brings things in perspective."

Kendra stayed with her search of who she was in relation to God and to those around her. Though she had always had a faith in God, she came to the conclusion that God had a claim on her life. Yet she still had a yearning to not miss any of life as a teenager. She was firm in her desire to follow God, but Kendra told Pastor Dan, "I don't want to be holy like you." There was a perception of an outward behavior for which she was not yet ready. As a teenager, there seemed to be so much of life still to explore.

At conferences and youth retreats, Kendra roomed with Laurie from Columbus, or Laurie E from Wooster. Bonnie no longer accompanied the group. Instead, she packed and sent microwave meals for Kendra to eat. Before each meal, Kendra would warm up her food in the kitchen while the other kids ganged up outside the dining hall waiting to eat. Separation during the pre-dinner hilarity was a price she paid to be independent and to be able to attend the retreats. After the meals, Kendra's laughter could be heard at the antics during the youth activities. She loved the freedom of being away from home and the chance to let loose with teenage humor.

Kendra avoided her stereotype of being super-spiritual, but as she finished her high school years, she remained aware of the testimony of her life before others. Mr. Buch, one of her high school math teachers, wrote a reference for Kendra's college application. He observed:

> *Kendra's Christianity is evident in her everyday life. … She has an integrity about her that is getting harder and harder to find in today's students. ... Kendra leads quietly by example. … Kendra's strength is her ability to know what is the right thing to do and then to follow through and do it. … Her*

*main weaknesses are health related. She has chronic health problems that take away her energy. She has made this potential weakness into a strength though. She never lets herself use her illness as an excuse.**

Kendra's first real relationship with a boyfriend began during her junior year in high school. Jim was a classmate and a casual friend who asked Kendra to their prom. They enjoyed each other's company and experienced the strong emotions of high school romance.

Throughout her senior year, Kendra and Jim spent a lot of time together. Kendra liked being one of the lucky girls who was dating. She was also pleased that part of their relationship included Jim's interest in attending the church youth activities with her and going on retreats.

Following high school graduation, Jim and Kendra separated. Kendra went to Grace College in Indiana and Jim attended a college closer to home. It wasn't just the physical separation that began to affect their relationship. By this time, Kendra had begun to solidify her commitment to the Lordship of Jesus Christ in her life. The pressures and struggles of her spiritual conflicts in high school were resolving into a desire to please God in all that she did. After she arrived at Grace College in the fall, she saw guys who were also growing in their faith and it focused her insight to the growing strain with Jim.

Pastor Dan recalled; "She wanted to maintain the

relationship and yet she was deeply committed to God. As Kendra's and Jim's relationship continued to grow, she saw Jim's spiritual growth centered on her growth. She wanted his growth to be independent. For Kendra, her relationship with God was more than living day-to-day, but was one where she wanted people to see Jesus living intimately in her. And she realized this was not where Jim was at."

Kendra broke up with Jim during the first weeks of college. She did not fall out of love with him, but she was learning to make spiritual decisions based on more than her emotions. In the following weeks, Kendra wrote a poem that reflected the sorrow and emotional confusion she felt.

To Jim
And Memories of Days Gone By

A curious touch, an inquisitive moment,
a gentle, warm, and friendly hug
was how it all began.

Trembling fingers reached up to
his shoulders as we danced the night away.
Magic was made that night, a feeling
I could not understand. But in that night,
that feeling, was something that could
never be taken away.

For in those days and weeks ahead, times
that I was confused, I found a soul

mate in those nights of lonely wanderings
along slow summer roads.

Somehow this friend that I had found
turned into something so much more.
For somewhere along these lonely
highways, I realized that it was
love that I had found.

A love so strong, so deep, so intensely
right, I could not fathom its
boundaries. Though one night along
the way we took a wrong turn, lost in a
town we didn't know. The "rightness"
went out of our relationship, never to
be grasped again. Slowly a wall
began to form between us and God.
I didn't know which side of the wall
I wanted to be on, the distinctions
grew fuzzy. I ignored God's prodding,
clinging to something I knew was not
right. Day after day, holding onto what
was slowly slipping away, I went a
bit insane. But somehow in the insanity,
I found solace in his arms.

Now that its all over, I've put a little
distance between us. I see God's loving

hand & the joy of doing what is right. Still in my
humanness, it's funny, but I miss the
insanity of it all & the solace in his loving arms.*

The decision to choose to follow God's leading was a pivotal point in Kendra's commitment to God and the changes that awaited her at college.

Chapter Four

KENDRA DID NOT HAVE A PERIOD OF REBELLION during her high school years. Lack of rebellion did not mean, however, that Kendra and her parents always understood each other. Communication tension rose at home during Kendra's senior year in high school as Bonnie, Terry, and Kendra tried to make decisions about college plans.

Kendra hesitated letting her parents know how badly she wanted to go away to Grace College in Indiana. She was very sensitive to Bonnie's fears for her protection and her need to have safe food. The Shultzmans were, in fact, pleased that Kendra was interested in Grace. They had many warm memories of their years there and still had friends in that area. Nevertheless, Bonnie and Terry wanted to talk through with Kendra how to handle safe eating concerns at a school away from home. Eating at the school dining hall was not an option because of the lack of control over ingredient and recipe changes.

When Bonnie tried to help Kendra work out ideas for eating at college, Kendra perceived it as her parents questioning her maturity and ability to handle her own life. It was difficult for Kendra to understand that her parents trusted her, but their wisdom saw that it was important to plan out the details of how to protect her health in a new environment. Kendra's youth wanted a more carefree approach.

This conflict in approaching the college decision confused Kendra and her parents. Kendra knew that she had proven herself to be mature and responsible regarding her health needs but she also wanted to honor her parents and their concerns. Sensing Kendra's hesitation, Bonnie and Terry concluded that she must be fearful of being on her own that far away from home. They also knew that she was concerned about the financial burden of attending college. Bonnie suggested that there were good schools closer to home. One school was within commuting distance, and at the other school, there was a family friend's home available for off-campus housing.

Terry could see how Bonnie and Kendra were each trying to alleviate the other's perceived fears. But he hoped that Kendra would choose Grace. "I thought it was time for her to be on her own. It was time for her to be away from us. I really wanted to see her learn to manage her own life."

Providence is God's care, through His choices and in His time, for what is His. The Shultzmans knew that they had been part of God's providence for Kendra's protection during her first eighteen years. At college, away from home, they would not be part of the active provision for Kendra's safety. After eighteen years it was hard to let go.

It was a season of growth for all three of them. Through prayer and communicating with one another, they finally reached agreement that Grace College was a good choice for Kendra. They felt good about her decision to attend Grace and had a sense of peace recognizing that she was under God's protection.

Kendra also grew in understanding of her parents' support and their sacrifice in letting her go, in order for her to continue to become a mature, independent young adult. Just before she left for Grace College, she wrote her parents a letter:

Dear Mom and Dad,

I guess I never realized how much I love you both until this year—how much a part of my life you are, until I discovered that you wouldn't always be with me. You wouldn't always be there to hold me when I am scared or to set me straight when I'd gone astray. You wouldn't be there to warn me against something that would bring me harm. I will have to make these decisions on my own now—so I started listening a little closer to what you were saying & tried to remember what it was you had told me in the past. But most of all, I started listening to my heart. I started taking action when that little voice would tell me to read my bible or to pray—even if it wasn't my scheduled time. I started to learn & take to heart what I was reading. I feel closer to God than I've ever felt before. For the first time in my life I feel He really *loves me*. I guess maybe that's just because I didn't *really* ever know Him before. I knew of Him & I believed with all my heart that He was God—but I never really *knew* Him. I guess now that you guys won't always be there, I have to listen to that little voice—that just might be the best thing that ever happened to me. I love you both so, so much—and I'm so scared to leave. But pray for me as I go that I will always listen to that voice!

I Love You!!

Kendra

P.S. No matter how old I get, in my heart I will always, always be your little girl.*

> *Look to the Lord and his strength; seek his face always. Remember the wonders he has done, his miracles, and the judgements he pronounced,*
>
> I Chronicles 16:11–12

As Kendra left for Grace College in the fall of 1990, she was determined to prove that she could be independent. She needed all of her resolute stubbornness to weather the first weeks on campus.

Laurie and Kendra had continued their correspondence throughout high school and roomed together at the summer youth conferences. They still considered each other best friends even after four years apart. Since both were planning to attend Grace College, they requested each other as roommates. Later, Laurie also asked another friend from Columbus to be a suitemate.

After their return from the Brethren National Youth Conference in August, Laurie and Kendra each found their room assignment letter waiting for them. They were assigned to a third floor suite. Bonnie and Kendra knew that the exertion of constantly climbing three flights of stairs would affect Kendra's asthma and cause her to wheeze.

During the same week, Kendra and Bonnie went out to the campus in Winona Lake to finalize arrangements with the school nurse, Joanne Taylor, regarding Kendra's medical needs. Mrs. Taylor agreed that the third floor room would increase the risk of health problems. She suggested that Kendra live on the main floor instead. Kendra hesitated because she knew Laurie was pleased with the third floor assignment. Mrs. Taylor proposed at least compromising on a second floor room.

When they returned to Ohio, Kendra called Laurie to make plans to switch their room assignment. After a long phone conversation, Kendra came away pale and worn out. Laurie would not make the change to another room. She felt committed to the arrangements with the other suitemate. Laurie wanted Kendra to go ahead and make plans to be on another floor and they would continue their reunion at college by being dormmates instead of suitemates. Kendra said to her mom, "I don't understand why Laurie won't room with me."

Kendra felt abandoned instead of supported by her best friend. Laurie continued to have the suitemate she knew, while Kendra had the uncertainty of moving in with a stranger. The rooming disagreement jeopardized their friendship. Neither Kendra nor Laurie had the skill or insight to talk through their confusion and maintain their relationship. The tension between them over the rooming decision did not resolve during their freshman year. Later Laurie said, "I never, ever wanted there to be any problems."

Kendra's personal choice to make the best of things and not complain served her well as she began her freshman year. She did not allow her reaction to negative circumstances get in the way of what was right and good in her life. Her decision to come to Grace was to prove that she was prepared to take control of her life, and she was determined to persevere.

Before college started, Kendra had already paid the price of a friendship to do what was necessary to stay at the college of her choice. On the first day at college, she began to pay the second price of assuming responsibility for her health.

At a small school like Grace, a great deal of the casual social life happens in the cafeteria as students met each other. Kendra was excluded from this casual dining atmosphere since she could not eat the cafeteria food. She felt too awkward to hang out in the dining hall if she didn't eat there. Just like at junior high school, she remained sensitive to all of the curious questions that would assail her about the food she wasn't eating.

Kendra received permission to cook her meals at a kitchen in a residence for retired missionaries which stood at the edge of campus. She stored her prepared meals in a refrigerator in her room and re-heated them in a microwave when needed. This need to have a separate eating arrangement was not going to stand in the way of enjoying her college experience.

Kendra joined the other freshmen in becoming familiar with the campus and its traditions. Since there were several social events during the early weeks, Kendra thought ahead to any areas of difficulty and she made choices necessary to protect herself from an allergic reaction to food substances. Kendra had the support of Joanne Taylor in making sure her stand for independence could proceed.

The freshmen were invited to get to know one another at Fireside gatherings in local faculty homes. Mrs. Taylor made sure that Kendra's invitation was to the Fireside in her own home. She then prepared a food buffet that included plenty of options for

Kendra so that Kendra would be free to eat casually along with everyone else there.

Later, there was the fun-filled evening of "initiation" for freshman when upperclassmen pulled pranks. Kendra made the decision to not participate in the evening. In the midst of hilarity, it would be difficult to explain that the spraying whipped cream had to be kept away from her.

After the initial disappointment of switching rooms, Kendra relaxed and enjoyed her new roommate, who became a great companion for easing into college life. Her name was Dayna, and she was already a sophomore. The two enjoyed great stories and laughter together.

Sunday afternoons became their special time to hang around their dorm room and laugh at each other's stories. Kendra introduced Dayna to the Eagles and Eric Clapton which were her favorite albums that year. Kendra's sense of humor also helped Dayna laugh at herself and put into perspective some tough issues affecting her.

On her part, Dayna tried to get Kendra to come over to the cafeteria and hang out, but Kendra felt she would appear out of place there. Dayna did make sure that Kendra had a chance to meet lots of new people. One of the fall traditions at Grace is *Rip Your Roommate* weekend where roommates fix each other up with blind dates to spark some social life on campus. Dayna knew that Kendra was making the decision to break up with her high school boyfriend so she wanted to make sure that Kendra participated. She set Kendra up with three blind dates.

One of the dates was with a junior art major named Don, who sat next to Kendra in her psychology class. Kendra and Don had a great evening. They found that they could talk about anything, that they both had a great sense of humor and sensitive natures. They began to spend more time together, often hanging out at the Art Building.

Kendra found a friend with whom to share some of her mealtimes. Leslie lived in the dorm and also had to avoid many foods. They were isolated from the camaraderie of the cafeteria, but they enjoyed each other's companionship. Leslie recalled, "We talked a lot as we cooked our meals, because we both understood what it felt like to be different."

Sometimes they would talk about heaven and what it would be like there. By the time they were in heaven and eating the feast presented there, they would have a perfect body. Much time and laughter was spent on deciding exactly which foods they were looking forward to eating at that feast.

They also talked about dreams. Leslie told Kendra about a couple of dreams she had about heaven and of how difficult it was to describe the beauty and peace she felt in those dreams. The dreams were so real to Leslie that in each dream she had wondered if she had actually died or if it was the Rapture—the taking of believers to meet Jesus Christ on His return to earth.

College students feel that they are immortal and don't often speak of heaven and death. But Leslie and Kendra shared the understanding that their medical problems placed their lives in danger and they were sensitive to the reality of death.

Dayna and Kendra continued to enjoy their Sunday afternoon time but by the end of the year they had drifted apart. Kendra was spending all of her extra time with Don. He had become her best friend.

When Kendra returned to campus for her sophomore year she knew that she had made the right decision to push for more independence in her life. Campus life, both in its freedoms and its responsibilities, merged well with her growing maturity.

The highlight of sophomore year for Kendra was the gift of friendship with two women, Brooke and Tracy. Brooke was a friend in the dorm, and Tracy was a friend of Brooke. The three girls spent hours together talking, laughing, sharing clothes, trying out different styles and double and triple dating. Kendra fixed Tracy up with Jeff who was a friend of Don. For one grand date that year the three friends and their dates rented a limousine and were escorted in style for the evening.

They all shared a love for music and played their favorite songs for each other. Kendra still had her picture from high school showing her in front of her poster of Michael W. Smith. She really liked his music.

Don and Kendra were established in a relationship that gave her security and a chance to love. Don was a great encourager. He supported Kendra's efforts toward a normal lifestyle. At Christmas, he gave her a membership in a local health center to increase her endurance with aerobic exercise.

Kendra controlled her allergies and health well at college. She made two visits to the Emergency Room, but each time the Emergency Room staff was able to stabilize her reaction. During the second semester of her sophomore year, Kendra marked a milestone towards normalcy. She started to eat in the cafeteria at times. Kendra wrote her parents in a letter, "Eating salads in the cafeteria is going OK. It's fun to get to talk to everyone at supper. I haven't had any problems with anything, yet."*

Kendra felt the need to continue to expand her options in life. She and Don even tried a few restaurants. The restaurants were usually Chinese which used oil and broths instead of butter in preparing the food. Kendra felt that she was reasonably prepared to choose her food carefully and ask adequate questions of the ingredients. She usually asked about the rice or salad. At times, though, she was tempted to try more variety.

Bonnie and Terry were concerned that Kendra did not understand the complexity of processed foods.

Kendra taste-tested each new item by briefly touching it to her tongue. An itching or tingling reaction indicated the need to avoid that food. However, with the more processed foods, there was a delayed reaction and Kendra sometimes had eaten more of the food before she realized she needed to avoid it. At times, Don tasted the food before Kendra to see if he could taste any butter or cheese in it.

Bonnie and Terry felt that eating in the restaurants was a great risk. There was no control over ingredients. They remembered the times in Africa where Kendra got sick simply because food was set down where cheese had previously been. They continued to stress to her the importance of being careful.

By the end of her sophomore year, Kendra had chosen Psychology and Business as a double major to focus her skills and her desire to work in helping others. Terry liked the strong individual Kendra was becoming as she matured. He considered her choice of major a wise decision. "She could understand other people's feelings and be compassionate. At the same time, she could also tell people what to do."

Kendra went home for the summer well satisfied with her liberty at college and looking forward to her junior year. The close supportive friendships with Brooke and Tracy gave her the security of acceptance by others. And, she was in a love relationship with Don that grew stronger as the months went by.

Chapter Five

WHEN KENDRA RETURNED TO WOOSTER in the summer of 1992, she and Laurie E attended some of the youth activities at church. The high schoolers enjoyed seeing the youth "alum." Kendra had a reputation as an encourager among the younger girls. "The conversation would be about you, not about her. She would make you feel better," recalled Sandy, one of the student leaders. Sandy's sister, Nikki, learned from Kendra that summer. "I knew that Kendra was trusting God. I could tell by just looking at her that she knew He was in control and was trusting God for everything."

Aaron Shultzman was in the high school youth group. Like Kendra, he did not seek out a leadership role for himself but supported others from behind the scenes. He had food allergies when younger, but not as severe as Kendra's. The youth members never heard either Kendra or Aaron complain about their food limitations. If the group went to a fast food restaurant that Aaron couldn't use, he would quietly go over to another and bring his food back to join them for the meal.

Robyn remembered hearing only once about the ongoing difficulties the Shultzmans had with food allergies. When Aaron was about seven or eight, a Sunday evening service was devoted to the congregation sharing what they were looking forward to in heaven. Aaron Shultzman stood up and proclaimed, "No allergies."

The youth group had established more focus since Kendra's and Laurie's high school years. Aaron and his peers had made a commitment to participate in a major project. The youth developed a program using Michael W. Smith's musical, ***The Big Picture.**** Kendra went to watch her brother in a performance.

The high schoolers had begun the project the previous fall, first studying the music and the message. The main characters were a group of teenagers going through a traumatic time after a car accident killed one friend and injured another. The story line and music presented God's providence as always being over each life, even if one didn't understand God's choice of allowing tragedy to touch young lives.

Pastor Dan understood the way the message of a performance would become personal for the individuals participating. He tried to prepare the group in recognizing the relationship of the musical to the reality of life. Even though teenagers tend to think of themselves as immortal, death does happen to people they know.

Just as the group was beginning to study the musical, two youth members were injured in a car accident returning from a retreat. Then a popular girl in the local high school committed suicide. The youth were shaken by these events and began to recognize the limits of their mortality.

By the summer of 1992, they had been performing the musical for six months for churches throughout the area. At every single performance there was someone in the audience who came up to share with them about a traumatic event which had evoked questions and confusion like those described in the musical. Pastor Dan observed that the youth were shaken by this maturing reality that life really was a matter of living and dying.

Over the summer, the youth group was taking a break in their performance schedule. The final performance was scheduled for November 15, 1992 in front of their home congregation at the Wooster Grace Brethren Church. It was originally set for September but was postponed in order to be part of the dedication month of the new building being completed for the church.

At first, the youth groaned at having to maintain performance readiness an extra two months. However, they were learning in the youth group to develop a servant's heart. If it was more helpful for the church to have them perform for the November dedication, then they were glad to comply. The summer months became a respite and the group used the time to create a new stage set to complement the increased facility at the new building.

Kendra used her summer break in a different way. Over the course of this summer, she and her parents were becoming friends on a more equal basis. After allowing Kendra to work through her need for increased independence, Bonnie and Terry were beginning to appreciate their daughter as an adult. They entertained Tracy, Jeff and Don in their home and liked the emerging relationships. In addition, Laurie E and Saralyn continued to drop by for visits. Bonnie and Terry sensed that these young adults were including them in their circle as friends, not just as Kendra's parents, and that these friendships would continue in the future.

Even though Kendra had such close friends, she still did not confide fears about her health with any of them. Brooke, Tracy and Kendra often spent long afternoons or evenings together covering any topic that came to mind. As they laughed and talked and tried on clothes, Kendra would sometimes quietly take a break and use her inhaler or take some medication. But it was understood that Kendra did not choose to talk much about this part of her life.

It continued to be with Bonnie alone that Kendra shared her very deepest fears. Kendra sensed that her health was deteriorating and it scared her. She questioned her mom. "If I am like this at twenty, what will I be like at thirty?" One evening, Bonnie and Kendra sat at the edge of their pool watching the setting sun. Kendra asked her mom, "What do you think heaven will be like?" Kendra was pensive and listened closely to her mom as she shared her answer. Later, Kendra told Brooke that she was really comforted by her mom's insights on heaven.

Kendra never spoke of her health concerns with her dad. But as Terry watched her struggling to breathe at times, he wondered if she would have a full life. Terry thought that if Kendra and Don got married they might move to a different climate where Kendra could breathe more easily.

Kendra had a visit with a cardiologist over the summer who gave her heart a clean bill of health. But because of Kendra's many questions about her health, the cardiologist suggested that she might seek a second opinion from another allergist. Kendra and Bonnie were later counseled by another physician that this second opinion probably wasn't necessary and the appointment was canceled.

At her annual visit to her regular allergy specialist later in the summer, Kendra wanted to speak to her doctor about some of her concerns. However, the day came and went without her taking the opportunity to ask for answers. His office was busy, and Kendra did not want to presume to ask him for more of his time to answer her questions. She had tears in her eyes after her examination as she was getting dressed and said to her mom, "I didn't get to ask him." In this case, her nature to always put others first worked against a very real need in her life to address her fears.

This intense period of concerns about her health continued for several weeks over the summer. Kendra turned to poetry to work out her feelings. Her feelings this time were not of love or hurt, but fear of her mortality:

> Pounding, Pounding
> I hear the rhythm in the night
> Searching for a place to hide
> Yet no shadow bids me stay
> I climb up tower stairs
> And run through stony corridors
> yet still I hear the pounding
> of the hoofs throughout the hills.
> He's ever riding, ever riding
> Holding shield and lance so high
> Echoing out through hills and valleys,
> "But my child, the time 'tis nigh"...
>
> *He risked His life for us, He*
> *died in the battle to save us,*
> *and yet look how we run from*
> *him, how ironic.*
>
> —Kendra Shultzman*

Later in the summer, Bonnie showed her own fears for Kendra's health. They attended the wedding of Heidi, Kendra's long-ago friend from Africa. At the catered reception, Kendra wanted to try one of the rice dishes being served. Bonnie tried to tell Kendra "No," and added, "Until you get a butter attack, you are not going to understand," but Kendra made light of her mom's concerns. Later Kendra glanced over and saw her mom crying. She asked "why?" Bonnie just shook her head, not wanting to get into their differences again over safe eating habits.

Kendra seemed to put her health fears behind her as she headed back to Grace College for her junior year. Pursuing her desire to focus on God, proceeding in her choice of a college major, and promising her life's love all merged at the beginning of Kendra's junior year.

Kendra was rooming with Brooke, and Tracy was the counselor on their floor. Brooke and Kendra agreed to be Growth Group Leaders and guide the spiritual life of the girls on their hallway. This group met weekly and studied together how to deepen their faith and apply it to their daily lives. Sometimes the group got silly, but Kendra, instead of enjoying the silliness as she usually did, kept drawing the group back to their study. Kendra's spiritual commitment had become serious business, and though she loved to laugh, she wanted each member to really consider letting Jesus Christ be at the center of all that they did and thought. In mid-November the Growth Group talked about heaven and Kendra shared with them her excitement about it.

During the fall, Kendra learned that she had been selected as a Peer Counselor on campus. This honor was a recognition of her maturity and a selection to be a role model for others. Kendra also knew by now what she wanted in her future and she described it in a poem to Don.

My Dream

My dream is to live out
contentment, to laugh, to love,
and to give.
To experience everything life
offers at the moment, to reach
out and grab opportunity.
To be filled with love from
God, family, and friends. To
rejoice in the good times. And
in the bad, to hold on to the very
foundations of life, and to be
sorrowful.
My dream is not to seek after
material things that can burn or be
taken away, but to seek after
those things which will last forever:
love, righteousness, holiness, and
sacrifice.

> My dream will take a lifetime
> to fulfill. It will not always be
> easy – but it will bring Glory to
> God my Father and fill my soul
> with contentment. Will you join
> me in my dream?
>
> —Kendra Shultzman*

Her dream included Don as her partner. In October, 1992, Don invited Kendra for a drive over to Lake Erie. There they ferried to an island. Don had previously planted clues for a treasure hunt throughout the island. At the end of the trail, near a pier, Kendra found a key. Don handed her a miniature treasure box. When she used the key to open it, she found an engagement ring! On bended knee, Don proposed to her and Kendra accepted!

When they returned to campus that evening their engagement literally rang the bells of Grace College. The campus tradition was to ring the tower bells to announce the arrival of a newly engaged couple. Announcements posted by friends during their absence invited all to a congratulations party. Friends greeted them on the outdoor patio.

Kendra was embarrassed by all of the attention but beamed with pleasure in showing off her ring. She enjoyed the excitement of others at her good news but her conversation was punctured by coughing.

Kendra, on this most exciting day of her life, was experiencing some respiratory stress after her long day.

Kendra called her parents to let them know of her engagement. Don had already asked their permission the previous summer to seek their daughter's hand in marriage. The Shultzmans could not have been happier. Bonnie was so delighted that her daughter had found someone who treasured her for the precious person that she was. Aaron enjoyed Don's company around the house. It was like having a big brother there. Terry liked Don and felt from his visits to their home that he was going to be a great friend. Terry, using his wry Shultzman humor, summarized his response, "Don was taking my little girl away from me. But I'd be pretty disappointed if someone didn't do that. I thought that Don was an excellent choice and they were good for each other."

It was an exciting time in Kendra's life. She and Don took many pictures of each other, trying to capture on film the emotions that they felt toward each other. Tracy and Brooke, too, were engaged. The conversations in the dorm began to focus on the specifics of wedding plans and marriage. The girls laughed at the reality that in the future it would not just be the three of them getting together, but there would be little ones clinging to them and trying to interrupt the conversations. Kendra spoke of her fears of being left behind. The youngest of the three, she would remain at Grace for at least a year after they left. She could not imagine herself without them.

As Kendra's life at college moved forward in faith and love, Bonnie began to prepare an engagement announcement to go in the Wooster, Ohio newspaper. She also helped Aaron get ready for the final performance of ***The Big Picture***. The new church building was complete, and the Wooster Grace Brethren congregation was finally going to see a performance of the musical that their youth had been presenting to others over the past year.

In the week prior to the performance, Bonnie had two different dreams about Kendra. They were tense dreams that evoked a lot of fear. In years past, Bonnie had other significant dreams that related to people she knew, including her own mother. Bonnie knew that she was worried about Kendra's health. Finally, at the end of the week, on the day of the performance, Bonnie called Kendra and told her of her dreams and concerns. She received Kendra's assurances that everything was fine and not to worry.

The final performance of ***The Big Picture*** was presented on Sunday evening, November 15, 1992. The congregation was awed by the quality of the performance and the maturity of the students presenting it. The youth were very gratified with the response of their home church. They were glad that the parents in the church could see them as more than just pizza eating, fun loving kids. The audience sensed how the message of God's providence had worked its way into each of their hearts. Bonnie found that the musical reminded her of God being in control and carrying out His plan in young lives. She spoke with a close friend after the performance. "Since there are so many students from Aaron's school in the musical, it is too bad it can't be used in some way at the high school."

This performance ended the project commitment for the youth. They had a high level of emotion and pleasure. They had performed before 1550 to 2000 people in the last twelve months. As a youth group, they probably had more perspective of life and death than any of the other youth groups in recent years. But no one in their home church had come up to them after the performance to relate how the message of this musical had been a reality in their life.

Chapter Six

On Monday evening, November 16, Brooke, Tracy, and Kendra gathered together for a long overdue session of fun. Their class assignments kept them busy and what little free time they had was usually spent with their fiancées.

When Kendra got excited she stood on her bed and stomped her feet. This night she stomped on the mattress and giggled as she talked about the image she had of Don and her being happy as a couple. The three young women promised that even though it was hard to get time together now, they would not lose contact after they had all gotten married.

They decided to try on different nail polishes and compare the results. As each different color dried on their fingernails, they gave their opinion of it. Kendra usually reacted to new things slowly. She wasn't sure that she liked the one brown-tone polish. She decided to put off her opinion of it until she could see it in a different light. The three of them stayed up laughing and talking until 1:30 A.M.

On Tuesday morning, November 17, Kendra sat cross-legged on the floor in front of the mirror. She slowly began fixing her hair. She called out to Brooke in the bathroom, "I had this weirdest dream last night." Brooke glanced out of the bathroom and could see the concern on Kendra's face.

"What was it about?"

"I had a dream that I died, and no one could see me but I could see them. I could see my mom. … She tried to talk to me … I feel really confused." Brooke felt the tension in Kendra's voice. She tried to lighten the mood with a laugh.

"You mean like you were there but no one could see you?"

Kendra answered, "Yes," and continued slowly getting ready for chapel. There was none of the normal morning chatter that usually filled the room. It was an odd contrast to the lightness of their time the night before.

After the girls left the dorm and got into Tracy's car, Kendra's mood changed. She was no longer distraught. Actually, she became exuberant like the night before. "I am going to ride in the front today," she laughed as she jumped into the car. Brooke and Tracy glanced at each other and smiled. Each of them had their habits, and one of Kendra's was to always climb into the back for the ride to campus. Kendra held out her hand and studied her polished nails. She turned towards Brooke and said, "You know, I think I do like this brown polish after all."

Following the chapel service, Don and Kendra walked across campus to get their mail. Kendra saw Leslie, her former meal partner. Instead of her usual "Hi," Kendra grabbed Leslie's long naturally curly hair and turned to Don. "This is what my hair is going to look like when it all grows out." Kendra then continued to encourage Leslie to stay and talk instead of running off to class. Leslie recalled, "...usually I said 'Hi' to Kendra and she would say 'Hi' back, but she grabbed me and it was like she *had* to talk with me. And I was in a hurry to get to class and she was like 'Talk with me for a minute.' It was 10:27 because it was right after chapel." It was unusual for Kendra to be so forward. Their friendship had become casual rather than close and they hadn't really talked in several weeks.

Later, Kendra met Don at the library to study. Instead of working, she spent her time whispering to him about her dream. He was her best friend, and she told him everything. He understood how this dream of death disturbed her. An acquaintance overheard some of their conversation. She thought to herself, "It is almost like she is telling him good-bye."

At 3:30, Brooke got a call from Kendra. "Brooke—guess what? I checked and we can schedule Growth

Group tonight. The other dorm meeting is going to be short so it won't conflict. I'm so glad. I'll take care of it all and write some notes to the members so that they will know to come. I really want us to meet tonight."

During supper, Kendra sat with Don's art group in the cafeteria. She listened in on their conversation and helped herself to some rice from Don's plate. The art students were trying to come up with a concept from three words. Kendra called out "Life!" Don leaned over and gave her a hug.

"That's right Kendra, you are life!" Following dinner she hurried back to her dorm.

An aerobics class was held every Tuesday and Thursday evening in the old Dining Hall on the first floor of the dorm. Kendra rushed into her dorm room to change clothes. The music was already blaring for the exercise time when Kendra ran down the stairs. Normally, she and Brooke sought out the back corner of the class to do their exercise. When Kendra got there this night, Brooke had found a space at the back, but the only opening for Kendra was way up front.

Kendra took the spot and started her exercising. Those in the front rows tended to work harder during the class. They knew everyone behind them could see how well they were doing. Brooke was a little concerned for Kendra as she watched her workout. Kendra stopped three different times to use her inhaler. She had told Brooke before, that when the weather was cold outside and she came into the warm dorm, it bothered her asthma. But Brooke knew that Kendra must feel okay, or else she wouldn't have even come to aerobics.

Finally, Kendra appeared to realize that she was overdoing it. Brooke watched her as she left the class. "Kendra's probably getting a drink of water," she thought.

A minute later, Kim, the Residence Director, came into the aerobics class and told Brooke, "Kendra needs to go to the hospital."

Brooke ran out the double doors and glanced up the stairway to her left. Kendra was just coming back down the stairs, scratching her hands. As Brooke raced up the stairs to help Kendra she noted, "This has to be a food allergy, not asthma, if she is feeling the need to itch."

Brooke met Kendra at the landing and helped her to the first floor lounge. Kendra was gasping for breath. "It's … never … been … this … bad … before. … It … was … something … I … ate. … I … can't … breathe. I … need … an … ambulance. I think … that … I … am … going … to … die."

Brooke ran to the counselor's room in the hallway. Kim was on the phone informing the college nurse that Kendra needed to go to the Emergency Room. Hearing from Brooke how desperate Kendra sounded, Kim ended the conversation and called 9-1-1.

Brooke rushed back to Kendra. She held a wet towel to her face and felt glad to be doing something to help her. Kendra kept patting Brooke's hand that held the towel, as if it felt good to her. Brooke noted that even though Kendra was having trouble breathing, she wasn't panicked. There was no fear evident.

Brooke kept running to the lounge window to see if the ambulance was there yet and then running back to Kendra. Kendra's color was really bad. Then Kendra suddenly lost all her color. A few minutes later the EMTs rushed in and took over. Brooke was held back and kept out of the way while the squad members fought to gain a pulse and respiration from Kendra. Brooke struggled with her anger to lash out at some of the students standing around who were saying that Kendra had just passed out. She knew that it was much more serious than that. The EMTs called into the hospital that they were about to transport an asthma attack victim.

Don arrived as Kendra was wheeled out to the squad. A campus security guard had informed him that Kendra was being taken to the Emergency Room. While driving to the dorm he kept thinking, "Kendra is having an allergy attack." He was prepared to see her gasping for air, "but instead they were rolling her toward the ambulance pale and still. Her hands and face looked like shaded snow."*

Terry Shultzman answered their phone about 6:35 P.M. It was Joanne Taylor, the Grace College nurse, calling from the hospital. She told him that Kendra had some problems and was on the way to the Emergency Room. Aaron was working on the computer and overheard the conversation. He understood that Kendra was going to the hospital, but it didn't seem that serious. He kept working. Terry handed the phone over to Bonnie because the ER needed a summary of Kendra's medications.

When the squad arrived at the hospital, the Shultzmans learned that when the EMTs had arrived at the dorm, Kendra had had no pulse and was in full cardiac and respiratory arrest. Bonnie was crying and praying as she heard the news. She stayed on the phone as Joanne kept updating information. Finally, Joanne called out, "They have a pulse!" Joanne and Bonnie were optimistic that maybe now Kendra had responded and was going to be okay.

When Terry heard that it had taken 45 minutes of CPR and intervention to reestablish Kendra's pulse and breathing, he considered that Kendra's life might be over or that Kendra would recover but with neurological damage. He struggled with the hope that he had misunderstood and Kendra would recover. But he had a heavy heart from that minute on.

While maintaining phone contact with the hospital, the Shultzmans went out to their garage to use the cellular phone in their car. They began to alert others of Kendra's emergency and to start prayer chain networks through the church. Bonnie arranged for a substitute for her classroom and they called Aaron's teacher. Terry's mother was asked to alert the relatives to the emergency. The Shultzmans had made previous arrangements for a pilot friend to transport them to Winona Lake, Indiana if there was ever an emergency. Bonnie contacted the pilot and told him that the flight was now necessary.

Even with the return of cardiac function, Kendra remained in a coma. During the early evening hours the hospital staff was watching for Kendra's body functions to resume. At last they felt that Kendra had stabilized enough for the Shultzmans to break off phone contact and to come and be with her. At 9:30 P.M. Bonnie took off from the Wayne County Airport in the small airplane. Aaron and Terry immediately started their four hour drive to Indiana.

On campus, Chaplain Roger Peugh went to the cafeteria commons to inform a party of several hundred students about Kendra's emergency. The students chose to end their party and moved off by themselves to pray.

Dayna was at another campus building watching the Comedy Night performance when the audience was informed of Kendra's illness. The program stopped and students began praying as the seriousness of Kendra's illness became apparent. Many of the students called friends on other campuses to inform them and ask for additional prayer support.

Bonnie arrived at the local airport at 11:30 and

was met by Joanne Taylor and Joan Darr, the Director of Nursing and a college classmate of Bonnie. The college nurse filled Bonnie in on the latest report of Kendra's condition. At the hospital, Kendra was not regaining consciousness. Don, Brooke, Tracy and others stood together praying. The waiting room was filled with those who were close to Kendra.

Bonnie, Don and Brooke spent the early hours of the morning visiting briefly at Kendra's bedside, praying and crying. When Bonnie first arrived, and said to Kendra, "I'm here," Kendra's eyes fluttered, struggling to open, and two quiet tears slipped down Kendra's cheeks. Since that brief response, there had been no other. Bonnie watched and considered that in heaven there would be no more tears.

Terry and Aaron arrived about 2:00 A.M. For the last several hours, Kendra's heart rate had been slowing down. Terry watched as the machine by Kendra's bed moved her chest up and down. Suddenly, a *Code Blue* was called. Bonnie asked the doctor if there was any hope. He said, "No."

At 3:35 A.M., Kendra's heart stopped and she died.

Chapter Seven

A FLOOD OF SHOCK AND SUPPORT flowed in during the early morning hours of Wednesday, November 18. Tracy's parents took Bonnie and Terry from the hospital to their home. The Shultzmans spent the next few hours making phone calls. Terry recalled, "We had never met these people before. We were very overwhelmed by the way people helped us out." The next morning the house began to fill with friends who wanted to be there for the Shultzmans.

This flood of shock and grief flowed past the Shultzmans and on to others who knew Kendra at Grace College and Wooster. The college community began to minister to the grief on campus. Initially, the campus administrators made sure that those closest to Kendra were informed personally of her death. Brooke, Tracy and Don had been at the hospital throughout the night. The college resident assistants made early dawn visits to others.

When Dayna first returned to her room after the Comedy Night performance was dismissed, she had thought that this emergency was like the other times that Kendra had needed to go to the Emergency Room. Dayna prayed for two hours as the word spread of Kendra's struggle at the hospital. She woke up at 4 A.M. and started to pray again. This time she knew in her heart that Kendra had died. She was sitting in her bed crying when her RA came at 6 A.M. to tell her.

Leslie also heard from her RA in the early morning hours. She was shocked and called others who were waiting to hear. Later that morning, Leslie glanced down at her watch. The time was 10:27. She realized that she had talked to Kendra just 24 hours ago and now she was gone. She began to cry as she realized the reality of Kendra's death.

The campus at large was informed during the morning chapel at 10:00 A.M. Chaplain Roger Peugh asked Joanne Taylor to give a report of the sequence of events of the previous night. He knew that hearing the details would help the students deal with some of their questions and also help them grasp the actuality of Kendra's sudden death. A college memorial service for Kendra was announced for one week from that day.

News of Kendra's death was shared with off-campus friends, and from community to community. The church community in Wooster was stunned. Just three days before the congregation had watched the dramatic musical about the providence of God allowing a special person to die. Suddenly, on Wednesday morning, came the news that Kendra, one of their own youth, had died while at college.

The calls from Wooster spread the word on to Kendra's friends away at other colleges. The phone startled Laurie E awake Wednesday morning. It was a double ring which meant an off-campus call coming through. Laurie hesitated to answer. An out of ordinary call usually brought stressful news. She was even more startled to hear her mom tell her that Kendra had died. Friends on her campus tried to comfort Laurie, but she quickly made plans to return to Wooster. "It was not going to sink in until I got home, because it is totally different at school. No one else knew her. They are still upset along with you, but it's not the same. Everyone was really good, but they couldn't do much."

Saralyn was in the middle of exam week at her college. She returned to her dorm room on Wednesday after taking her worst final exam. When she answered the phone and realized that her mom was calling her mid-day she thought that it was weird. Phone calls normally came during off-rate hours. Her mom said, "I have some bad news," and told Saralyn of Kendra's death.

Saralyn's first reaction was disbelief, thinking briefly that maybe her mom was making a bad joke.

She sat in her room that day dazed and crying while her friends tried to offer her comfort. But none of them had just lost one of their best friends. She looked at the card on her desk that she had purchased that morning to save for Kendra's birthday. Then Saralyn glanced down and realized that when she had gotten dressed in the dark that morning, she had put on only black clothes.

A sudden death leaves a family unprepared with funeral decisions. Time pressed against the Shultzmans to plan a service to honor the memory of their daughter while their mind and emotions were still numbed against the reality of her death. Bonnie and Terry made the decision to have Don be a partner in the planning of the memorial service. His loss of a fiancée was significant. He also helped them select the grave site. The calling hours were scheduled for Friday evening and the memorial service and burial were planned for Saturday, November 21.

The Shultzmans made two decisions regarding the service. Kendra's best friends from college, her fiancée Don, and friends Brooke and Tracy, were to be given places of honor; and ***The Big Picture*** would be a central theme of the service. When Bonnie spoke with Dan Travis the day after Kendra died, she said, "The only thing that has been going through my mind is the musical." The message of the musical, and the timing of the last performance, gave a framework for understanding that in God's providence, Kendra's death was not a surprise nor an accident.

Thursday and Friday were spent going through family photos. A video train of photographs set to music was planned for the memorial service to show Kendra as she grew up. The Shultzmans also developed a poster board of pictures to be displayed during the calling hours at the funeral home. There were poignant moments even in their pain, as family and friends went through the pictures and remembered funny stories from Kendra's life.

By Friday evening, four days to the hour after their world came apart with a phone call, the Shultzmans were standing in a receiving line at the funeral home waiting to greet and be comforted by those who were also seeking comfort. Hundreds waited in the line that stretched through the rooms and out into the parking lot as friends from church and the community came to work out their sorrow together. Those waiting to speak to the Shultzmans spoke quietly to one another. It was a visiting time for them until they inched their way forward and tried to come up with words to offer to Bonnie, Terry and Aaron.

Kendra's death had taken her from life to *Life*. She instantly came into the presence of the living God, surrounded by holiness, who welcomed her with love and joy. For those left behind, and not yet on the same journey, Kendra's death left a different setting. Those present this evening wished that the need for these calling hours had not arisen. But the time was here, and even if there were no words, their presence conveyed that they shared the shock and sorrow brought by Kendra's death.

Amish builders, who Terry had worked with at the lumber company, lined up with Kendra's friends who had returned home from their colleges. One of Bonnie's third grade students grabbed her teacher and hugged her, not having any other words to say. Friends of Aaron, from school and church, stood silently.

Just before those waiting reached the head of the line, they had an opportunity to read a poem which Don had penned in the days since Kendra's death.

The Fragile Flower

by don swartzentruber

we stood together
i now stand alone
my fragile flower has died.

her premonition has fulfilled
the dream of immortality
frustrations that she could not speak
to the ones she left behind.

it seems especially cold at night
thinking of her body white
and
still
hoping she would awake
at least to kiss and say good-bye.

my promise of marriage
will stay on her hand
maybe it is beautiful enough God will allow
kendra to take it along
and she will thank me …
someday.

as my heart bleeds
i know
i will see her on the other side

God help me redeem the time.*

The next morning, Kendra's memorial service was scheduled for 11:00 A.M. Six days previously ***The Big Picture*** had been the first musical presented in the new building. Now, Kendra's was the first memorial service. The entire auditorium was filled as the video train of Kendra's photographs filled the screen and the music reminded people that Kendra was now free in her heavenly home.

Roger Peugh, the Chaplain at the college, spoke at the service. He shared that the verse *"Make me to know my end and what is the measure of my day"* (Psalms 39:4 KJV) was the framework under which Kendra lived. She lived her life for God and had learned to number her days. Chaplain Peugh expressed that the tension the congregation was feeling between joy for Kendra and sorrow and the questions they had about their loss of Kendra were both normal and appropriate on this day. The deep sense of loss at this moment was real, and those present needed to accept that there were questions about "why" for which there were no answers.

The Shultzmans had asked the youth chorus to sing at the memorial service. They stood and sang the song "I Hear Leesha" from ***The Big Picture***. In the musical, this was a song of grief and comfort following their friend's death. During this memorial service, the youth sang Kendra's name in place of "Leesha." The song helped them begin to understand that her death came within the providence of God. Nikki sang part of the song as a solo and looked at the Shultzmans as she sang, offering the song as the comfort the youth could share.

Pastor Bob Fetterhoff spoke to the one question which dominated at her "untimely" death. "Why?" He quoted from Isaiah "*... devout men are taken away and no one understands.*" (Isaiah 57:1b). He reviewed the right priorities which Kendra had chosen to make in her relationship with her God, her family and her friends.

The service ended with more video pictures of Kendra. The music playing in the background was one of Kendra's favorite songs—about meeting a friend again on the other side of death.

As Terry Shultzman escorted his wife to the limousine for the ride to the grave site, it was hard for him to grasp why there were so many at Kendra's service and why there was such a response to her death. "I know that all of our children are very precious to any parent, and I know when a person dies at an early age that a lot of people respond, but it seems … that it has been overwhelming." The limousine driver told Terry that he had been to 136 services and this was the second largest he had seen. The only other one that was larger was for the mayor of a city.

What was it that drew so many out to attend Kendra's service?. She was not a world famous celebrity. She did not hold any positions of leadership in her community or in her church fellowship. She was a twenty year old young woman going about the business of growing up.

Many came to the service to honor Kendra, recognizing that she had chosen to allow God's involvement in her daily life. Kendra's life was presented at the service as one who knew the uncertainties of her health, but also as one who chose to align herself rightly with God. Her life reflected the joy that came from God, not from perfect circumstances in the world. This right focus sustained her through the added burden of her health fears. Many in the congregation, having seen ***The Big Picture***, and then attending the memorial service, recognized their own need to acknowledge God as a living Presence, and Maker of choices in day-to-day life.

The Shultzmans returned to Grace College that same week for the college's memorial service. They heard additional remembrances from students about Kendra's quiet spirit and her joy of life. The students' remembrances focused on her exuberance and laughter, and the way she showed how to live life God's way.

The students on campus had worked out their grief in different ways. There were two general reactions. The first was, "We lost Kendra." This fellow student, who they knew and liked, was gone from their midst. The second reaction was, "It could happen to me." Joanne Taylor reported that it was not the women students who reacted most strongly, but the engaged men. They empathized with Don and wondered how they would go on when one's future plans were no longer secure.

For some who knew Kendra well, there were personal reactions of regret that they had not spent more time with her, and now the opportunity to do that was gone. For others who knew her less well, it was easier to distance themselves and begin again to think that death could not happen to them.

Kendra's death continued to touch others in the Wooster community, The high school youth at the Grace Brethren Church grieved for Kendra, but they also grieved for themselves. They understood their own immortality. If Kendra died, then so could they. Many recognized that being under God's care did not mean that He always made the choices which one expected. They realized again the uncertainties of life.

These thoughts of God had caused four youth who attended the youth group to give up their fence sitting attitudes, and to declare themselves prepared to acknowledge that God was living and had a claim on their life. They asked for God's forgiveness offered through the sacrifice of His Son, and invited Jesus Christ to be Lord of their life.

More impact on the youth in the community occurred in the week following the memorial service. While speaking with a teacher at the school, Bonnie explained how the message of ***The Big Picture*** had meant so much in trying to understand Kendra's death. The high school principal knew that many of the students were stunned and upset that someone they knew had died. He agreed that a voluntary assembly should be held as a memorial to Kendra and to help the high schoolers think through some of the grief that they were experiencing. The church youth group was invited to present ***The Big Picture*** at Kendra's former high school.

The memorial assembly at Triway High School was presented before a packed auditorium with kids standing in the aisles. Bonnie was given an opportunity at the beginning to address the students. She spoke of the impact that ***The Big Picture*** had on their family in trying to understand Kendra's death, and she concluded her remarks by saying, "My prayer is that God will teach all of us to number our days, that we may apply our hearts to wisdom." For the Grace Brethren youth, the unexpected performance at this local high school was another piece of the puzzle of how God was choosing to use Kendra's death in the life of others. The high school students' responses were very gratifying as they understood the message of God's providence.

Pastor Dan appreciated Terry and Bonnie Shultzman's openness to use a memorial assembly at the high school to present the gospel. He knew that from Kendra's perspective, she would have chosen that. "If she was going to die prematurely in the world's eyes, then she would want her death to be used as a tool to help draw others into the Kingdom."

For the first fourteen days following Kendra's death, the Shultzmans were carried along by the necessity of traveling from Indiana back to Wooster, making funeral plans, holding the memorial service, returning to Indiana for the Grace College memorial service, driving back to Ohio, and speaking at the memorial assembly at the high school. During this time there was a spiritual and emotional shock following Kendra's sudden death that wrapped a cocoon of numbness around them. God's grace soothed some of the emotions and made it bearable. Then suddenly, two weeks after Kendra died, the immediate demands on their time lessened and the shock was wearing off. Bonnie, Terry and Aaron were left with the raw pain of grief.

Chapter Eight

As the Shultzmans began to live with the heavy burden of grief, others tried to offer comfort through their words. Some words focused on Kendra. A member of Kendra's Growth Group from Grace College wrote: "I know the holidays must've been very hard. It's still hard for me to understand why God took Kendra to heaven but she was a very special Christian—that I do know."* Other words focused on the Shultzmans. "You have achieved such a wonderful accomplishment by raising a lovely young lady who was wise and self-assured and not handicapped by her 'illness.'"*

They valued every detail that they picked up from others. "It still jars me almost like a physical blow when I think of Kendra's death. She came into the mailroom the morning of the day she died and as usual I thought … 'what a lovely gal she is.' She was a reflection of her love for God and of the love and care and prayers and tears of loving parents."* "God gave

Kendra a special talent for joy even with all the restrictions in her life."* It was encouraging for the Shultzmans to know that others saw Kendra like they did.

As the Shultzmans went about the community completing necessary errands, they were surprised that even strangers, upon learning their name, would comment on having read and remembered the obituary. They were comforted that even these strangers were saddened by Kendra's death at such a young age. An acquaintance told Terry, "It has rocked the community."

Bonnie found that tears and laughter mixed as she struggled through her days. Even on the night of the memorial service she realized, "We laughed and we cried at the same time—I felt guilty for laughing, yet being able to laugh is part of the grief process." At home, Bonnie chose to bring up Kendra's name with "Remember when Kendra …" and the Shultzmans continued to laugh and cry together.

Terry, normally a reticent man at work, began to speak with those around him about his daughter. He sought their comfort and understanding at the trauma occurring in his life. Aaron was also quiet, but shared with Pastor Dan his struggles in missing Kendra. She was not only his sister but also his best friend. The youth group tried to stand by him and let him know they cared, even if he didn't feel like talking.

Bonnie experienced unexpected glimpses of insight and comfort in the midst of her days. There are many cloudy days in Ohio. One day there was a filtering of sun coming through the clouds. "I saw that and it just brought tears to my eyes. Kendra and I really had a lot of the same ideas—she really wanted to be where it was warm. When I saw that ray of sunshine, I thought, Kendra has done just that. She went where there is sunshine."

It was also comforting to know that there was an ongoing impact from Kendra's life and death. During Kendra's birthday week, Roger Peugh wrote a letter to her parents. "On Thursday, four men students gave testimony of their growing relationship with Christ, turning way from a life of emptiness and hypocrisy as Christians. ... We know that Kendra's death continues to have a sobering, teaching effect on our campus and for this we are deeply thankful."*

Some words and actions meant to comfort brought the recognition that few understood the grief that they were enduring. At times they needed a hug or a gentle recognition that this nightmare they were living would eventually be more tolerable. Instead, they found themselves isolated and left alone by others who didn't know how to be around those who are hurting.

Many trying to help the Shultzmans had no way to measure how long one grieved on the inside. "Those of us who know you and the faith that you have, know that you will find comfort in the Lord. … I guess what I'm trying to say is—that everyone knows you'll be all right for that reason."* The Shultzmans would eventually have some healing, but there were dark valleys to travel through on the way.

Some friends were anxious that the Shultzmans be able to put their grief behind them and get on with their lives. Many chose to speak of only ordinary, everyday topics with the Shultzmans. But for the Shultzmans there was not yet anything normal in their lives.

While Bonnie's heart was aching for Kendra's presence, her mind was struggling with "if only…". Bonnie had held the most responsibility of protecting Kendra's food supply through the growing up years. Bonnie had held the most fears about Kendra accepting that responsibility by herself at college. During the first year of grief, Bonnie spent a lot of time trying to sort out a series of "if only" ideas. "If only I had understood earlier her increasing fears for her health, if only…" It was difficult for Terry to watch Bonnie blaming herself for not protecting Kendra enough. "Bonnie is going through a time of 'if only I had done this … or that.' But Bonnie was a great mother. She shouldn't be faulting herself."

Bonnie's questions changed from "if only…?" to "what if…?" On the night Kendra died, the physicians spoke with the Shultzmans. But later during her grief, Bonnie wanted to ask additional questions of the physician who attended Kendra in her last hours. "That night is just a blur. I knew that there were a lot of kids there, but it is just a blur. I have a lot of very vivid memories. I probably wish that I had asked a lot more questions that night." Several months later, Bonnie tried to speak with the attending physician, but he did not respond to her request to talk. She wanted answers to her "what if…?" What if the doctors had given Benadryl early on, right after Kendra was resuscitated? What if the doctors had understood it was a food allergy and not an asthma attack? What if she had been transferred to another hospital? What if…?

Joanne Taylor, the college nurse, found comfort during her own grief from some of the exceptional circumstances surrounding the evening Kendra died. She shared her comfort with Bonnie. Joanne knew that the ambulance and EMTs had arrived at Kendra's side quickly and were able to start CPR soon after she had lost consciousness. Kendra arrived at the Emergency Room just at shift change so there were two physicians present to help her. In addition, the hospital had sent staff over to an Internal Medicine physician's home to watch his children so that he would be free to also come to the Emergency Room. Kendra's pulse and blood pressure were stabilized soon after her arrival at the hospital. She believed that everything humanly possible was done.

Bonnie wanted more questions answered so that

she could also believe that. Was there some understanding of Kendra's medical problems that Bonnie had picked up from years of being Kendra's main protector that could have unlocked the key to Kendra's survival? Joanne shared Bonnie's frustration that in this particular occurrence, Kendra's allergic reaction happened more quickly and that she did not respond as before to medical intervention. Even with her unanswered questions, Bonnie acknowledged to Joanne, "It comes down to this was her time." They shared this comfort together.

An additional comfort that they could share together was Joanne's observation that there was no panic for Kendra. Even though her reaction moved quickly, she evidenced a calmness during that time. Joanne believed that Kendra was already entering the presence of God and had Jesus at her side.

During the long period of grief, the Shultzmans found that many of the cards and messages of sympathy they received did not result in the expected comfort. Especially difficult were some of the condolences quoting scripture. The cards gave scripture verses reminding them that Kendra was a Christian and therefore better off in heaven. Others tried to encourage the Shultzmans by pointing to their victorious future with Kendra in heaven. But these cards were countered by the present pain which they felt. The truth was correct but it did not minister to the heart that was hurting.

The Shultzmans loved Kendra and remembered her love of life. They wanted her to still be with them. Sometimes their feelings of grief, held against the truth of scripture, left the Shultzmans feeling guilty that the scripture which they loved did not at this time offer the expected comfort. The Shultzmans found that the heart and mind each needed time to heal in the midst of this hurt. Their emotional wound grew smaller in time, but did not completely heal. Though their comfort increased, the total healing will be completed when they also are home in the presence of God.

Bonnie and Terry found it was also hard in the beginning to draw comfort from God through prayer. When Kendra became ill and news traveled around the campus, students called their families and church prayer chains around the country. Bonnie said, "It is incredible to me—I've never heard of anyone else who had so many prayers offered." That recognition brought comfort. Yet it was countered with the recognition that even with all of those prayers, God chose to let Kendra die.

What was the effect of the prayers? How can one pray to God for comfort, when He didn't respond to prayers for her life? It takes a growing understanding and trust of God to recognize that while one is to earnestly communicate our desires through prayers offered, the answer remains in God's choice, in His providence.

During the week of the memorial service, there was great comfort from the songs of providence in ***The Big Picture*** but over the next year these same songs became bittersweet as specific questions troubled Terry and Bonnie. Providence to many means the loving hand of God providing "good" things in our lives. God's providence actually means that He acts in love and care in choices made for our lives. Yet, His choice was to let Kendra die. Terry and Bonnie struggled with anger and confusion toward God as they continued to try to understand why Kendra's death was God's choice. Their faith during grief was strained and stretched to trust a God who acted beyond their human understanding.

Many tried to comfort the Shultzmans by giving ideas of "why" Kendra died. Reasons offered to the Shultzmans to help answer their "why" included; *things like this just happen, eating the butter was just a accident, she is better off since she would be sick, it was worth it for Kendra to die because there are eight new believers now because of her death. Kendra had finished what God had for her.*

There were elements of truth in each of these reasons. Accidents do "just happen," and Kendra is better off in heaven with her new body and in the presence of the Lord. There is much to rejoice that there are eight new believers. God does have purpose and works planned for us. But these attempts at encouragement didn't offer a correct perspective of God.

If events "just happen," does that mean God is powerless in our everyday lives? Couldn't God have prevented this "accident?" Even if Kendra is "better off" in heaven, does that mean there was no more joy for her here on earth, or for others with her? Was there no other way for God to gain access to the hearts of the new believers than through Kendra's death? Chaplain Peugh had addressed this issue during the memorial service. "It is not a true equation that *If something good happens following her death* then it was *worth it all*."

The Bible is clear that God will accomplish the plans He has for each believer, and He will take that believer home, but scripture does not say that one is taken home to be with the Lord just as soon as those plans are accomplished. There are many elderly believers who need to accept diminishing control over their bodies and lives, while they wait for their numbered days to end.

If these direct, *easier* answers to why Kendra died were not acceptable, then the alternative for the Shultzmans was to struggle with their understanding of God and what it means to be under the providence of God. There was only partial comfort in knowing God may have been protecting Kendra from further serious health problems in the future. Terry said, "It was so hard for me to see Kendra restricted more and more. Maybe that was down the road for her, and God decided." But, Terry grappled with the fact that

God had allowed Kendra to have her allergies and asthma in the first place. So God's allowances for Kendra's life included the very allergy that contributed to her death.

These two ideas of understanding that God both allows pain and comforts our pain are described in Lamentations 3:32-33: *Though he brings grief, he will show compassion, so great is his unfailing love. For he does not willingly bring affliction or grief to the children of man.*

In his book **Trusting God**, Jerry Bridges wrote of this struggle. "Sometimes we come to the place where we do not demand of God that He explain Himself, but we try to determine or comprehend for ourselves what God is doing. We are unwilling to live without rational reasons for what is happening to us or those we love. We are almost insatiable in our quest for the *why* of the adversity that has come upon us."*

In the midst of grief, peace and trust are dependent on each other. The Shultzmans were slowly brought to the point of trust over emotions. Kendra did not die outside of the control of God, but was allowed to die within His capability to prevent it. "If we are to honor God by trusting Him, and if we are to find peace for ourselves, we must come to the place where we can honestly say, 'God, I do not have to understand. I will just trust You.'"*

Chapter Nine

AFTER THE INITIAL REACTION of anger and shock at Kendra's death, there was a growing recognition of God's hand of providence tenderly caring for Kendra in her sudden transition from life here on earth to life with Him in heaven. Joanne Taylor related to the college community at the announcement of Kendra's death: "[the] night before last, Kendra had a dream that she died, and she told two of her favorite friends yesterday. Kendra was prepared and tried to prepare her friends. She talked at supper last night with a friend of how she'd wanted to most be remembered. I think God truly prepared Kendra for her going home. I think we need to realize that every time we think of heaven doesn't mean God's preparing us for that day. But I think that God will prepare us when it's our time. And He did prepare Kendra for last night."*

In sharing their experiences surrounding Kendra's death, others recognized God's providence in also preparing them. Bonnie had the two troubling dreams in the week before Kendra's death, causing her to consider that something wasn't quite right. Brooke and Tracy had a long awaited time together with Kendra the night before she died. Dayna was awakened in the middle of the night and knew that this time Kendra had died. Saralyn awakened in the middle of the night and felt terrified. She thought that she must be very nervous about her exam coming up the next morning. Later, she realized that she had awakened at the exact time that Kendra died.

God's providence for one person becomes in part his providence for others. The choice He made in loving concern for Kendra also became choices affecting others. The providence of Kendra's death meant that the Shultzmans lost Kendra's future friendship. Don no longer had a fiancée. Brooke, Tracy and other friends no longer could project ideas of their children growing up to be friends. Aaron was now without his best friend and comrade-in-arms around their home.

For many of Kendra's friends, her death was their first experience with the loss of a friend. Laurie recognized that one never knows what life is going to hold. "She was engaged and going to graduate and all of those good things. You just don't understand. Not a day goes by that I don't think of her. It wasn't that I was afraid to die … but after she died I remember thinking I am not afraid if I die. I am not afraid."

Sandy found herself more aware of heaven. "I'm going to see her on the other side. She is going to be so much better—not afraid of what to eat. I don't need to fear anything or be upset because God has her now."

Laurie E had difficulty with the timing of Kendra's death. "She was getting the Peer Counseling that she wanted to do. And that has me scared, I mean like, when I have some dreams that are going to start coming through, am I going to be scared that I am going to die?" In addition, Laurie E realized that grieving takes unexpected twists and is not limited to the immediate time of death. "I still think that I need to grieve some more, but I can't trigger it. … It is settling in even more as time goes on. Like this summer. She used to always be there. We would go to church. She wasn't there to go with."

In the three years following Kendra's death there were a lot of *firsts* which brought the Shultzmans renewed recognition of her absence. There was Thanksgiving. There was Christmas. There was Kendra's birthday. There was Easter. There was the Spring Banquet at Grace College. There was Mother's Day. There was Brooke's and Tracy's graduation. There was Father's Day. There was Tracy's wedding. There was Kendra's class graduation. There was Brooke's wedding. There was Aaron's high school graduation. There was the birth of Brooke's baby.

There was life continuing to be lived by all who knew Kendra, only Kendra was no longer here to laugh and enjoy this life with them.

Terry and Bonnie found enjoyment through continuing relationships with some of Kendra's friends. Brooke became part of their extended family. Laurie E and Saralyn continued to visit. They attended the wedding of Laurie. They spent time with Don and his new wife.

Over time, Bonnie focused more on what Kendra gained from her "early" entrance to heaven, rather than what those grieving lost. "All those feelings I had about Kendra being shortchanged … marriage, children, travel. I am coming to understand that she has traveled in the blink of an eye; she has already done it. All these things she has ever wanted to do, all these foods she has ever wanted to eat. She has done it."

Bonnie found solace during these years in building up her understanding of what heaven is like, and growing in understanding of the *Life* that Kendra is now living. Part of Bonnie's soul yearned to move quickly on to that *Life* so that she could be reunited with Kendra. Bonnie continued to miss Kendra's laughter and companionship and the friendship that she and Kendra were just moving into in their shared adult relationship.

Bonnie found a gift in the area of writing poetry. The poems helped focus her thoughts and feelings and also communicated well with others who were experiencing similar grief in their lives. She continues to move slowly through her grief, and uses what she is learning to comfort others.

Kendra's death made Dayna realize that there is never a certainty of how much time there will be for a goal. She wrote a poem expressing her feelings at Kendra's death and what she learned:

For Kendra

When I think about the time I've lost,
My heart breaks in two.
I am trying to put into perspective why He has taken you.
My mind fills with questions and that never ending why.
And in the silence of those pounding thoughts,
I hear you whisper,
"But my friend, my time was nigh."
And suddenly I can feel you!
I feel you laughing that [contagious] laugh
of yours and I just have to join in.
You have become all that scares me
(in my sinful selfishness
of not wanting to leave what has become comfortable)
and you have become all that I hope and dream for. ...
To be with our Lord and Maker.
Because of you,
I have learned not to take anything for granted.
You are the essence of life!
You knew your destiny was done—
You, my friend, have won.*

There were other spiritual ramifications to consider. For Nikki, she realized that she was not afraid of her own death, but fearful for friends who didn't know God. If someone their age could die, then it would be really important to be sharing with her friends about God. Robyn felt a responsibility to share with friends how to know God, so that if they died young, they wouldn't feel like no one had told them.

Many of Kendra's peers came to a new recognition that God's providence determined how long they would live:

> *My times are in your hands.* (Psalms 31:15)
>
> *Man's days are determined; you have decreed the number of his months and have set limits he cannot exceed.* (Job 14:5)
>
> *Your eyes saw my unformed body. All the days ordained for me were written in your book before one of them came to be.* (Psalms 139:16)
>
> *Show me, O Lord, my life's end and the number of my days; let me know how fleeting is my life.* (Psalms 39:4)

Though Kendra seemed to have some growing hints that her days were numbered, the story of providence in Kendra's life was of how she chose to live those days. Kendra's life reflected life at its best. Kendra had a heart that turned to God at an early age. That is a gift. She chose as she grew not to turn that heart to rebellion. That was a choice. Because her heart stayed turned towards God and His choices for her, her life evidenced the fruits of the spirit: *...the fruit of the Spirit is love, joy, peace, patience, kindness, goodness, faithfulness, gentleness and self-control.* (Galatians 5:22a)

Kendra did not respond with complaints to what was imposed on her life. She responded with an attitude of joy towards God and enjoyment of others. As a young adult, Kendra was already making Godly choices with her life. She had chosen to become a disciple of the Lord Jesus Christ. She placed herself in a position under God's authority to use her life as He saw fit. She had a trust in God that His providence meant that she was under His care, willing to accept His choices made for her in His time.

Kendra recognized her growing focus in life. In the last year of her life she wrote a paper entitled *Impacting My World.* In it she concluded, "As I journey through life, I want to make an impact in people's lives. I want to show them that I care. I hope that's what I've done and what I will continue to do."*

The story of Kendra's journey ends here. But the story of the providence of God continues in the life of each of us. God gives to all of us the same freedom of choice to live life God's way and choose to trust God for His choices for our love and our care.

Oh How I Love You!

From the first time I saw you I loved you!
  You were a bundle of joy from the start.
You cooed, and snuggled, and wiggled, and cried,
  And I cuddled you close to my heart.

You were two and oh how I loved you!
  You had curls and eyes of blue.
You laughed and giggled, talked and sang,
  Till you charmed me through and through.

When you were four I especially love you!
  You travelled to places unknown.
Your life was different than most little girls,
  Yet your bright eyes and smile still shone.

You turned six and I dearly loved you!
  By then you had a brother of two.
You were sister, playmate, helper and friend,
  To a brother who dearly loved you.

You were eight and oh how I loved you!
  You were now a student in school.
You worked and laughed, played and ran,
  As the autumn days turned cool.

When you were ten I especially loved you!
  How close you'd grown to my heart.
You helped in the garden, and around the home,
  Always doing your part.

You turned twelve and I dearly loved you!
  You'd become a little lady by then.
You borrowed my clothes, and did your own hair,
  Went to slumber parties of friends.

You were fourteen and oh how I loved you!
  By then you'd become a teen.
You thought your own thoughts, and did your own things,
  Held your friends in high esteem.

When you were sixteen I especially loved you!
  You were lovely and full of grace.
You understood life, that few knew about,
  It showed in your beautiful face.

You turned eighteen and I dearly loved you!
  You'd become wise beyond your years.
You wrote about life—It was precious to you.
  You allowed Jesus to calm your fears.

You were twenty and oh how I loved you!
  You'd become engaged to your very best friend.
We didn't know, we couldn't know,
  Your life was soon to end.

You're with Jesus, and oh how I love you!
  He holds you in sweet embrace.
He smiles and says, "Oh how I love you!"
  As you see Him face to face.

—Bonnie Shultzman
In loving memory of Kendra*

END NOTES

Chapter One

Page 11, Jan Hastings, personal note, fall, 1992.

Pages 11–12, Kendra Shultzman, poem, second grade.

Page 15, Kendra Shultzman, *My Most Memorable Day*, essay, tenth grade.

Chapter Two

Page 21, Kendra Shultzman, *Paper On Adolescence*, October 26, 1992.

Page 22, Kendra Shultzman, letter, summer, 1986.

Chapter Three

Pages 28–29, Kendra Shultzman, *Paper On Adolescence*, October 26, 1992.

Page 32, Tom Buch, personal notes for college reference, 1990.

Pages 33–35, Kendra Shultzman, *To Jim—And Memories of Days Gone By*, poem, November 3, 1990.

Chapter Four

Pages 38–39, Kendra Shultzman, personal letter, 1990.

Page 46, Kendra Shultzman, personal letter, January 28, 1992.

Chapter Five

Page 49, ***The Big Picture***, Written by Andy Stanley, Music by Michael W. Smith, Copyright 1991, Word Music.

Page 53, Kendra Shultzman, poem, summer, 1992.

Pages 55–56, Kendra Shultzman, *My Dream*, poem, fall, 1992.

Chapter Six

Page 65, Don Swartzentruber, paper on *Kendra's Death and Poetry*, December 10, 1992.

Chapter Seven

Pages 74–75, Don Swartzentruber, *The Fragile Flower*, paper on *Kendra's Death and Poetry*, December 10, 1992 (written November, 1992).

Chapter Eight

Page 81, Rachel, letter, January 13, 1993.

Page 81, Jan Hastings, letter, November, 1992.

Page 81, Hyla Snider, note on card, November, 1992.

Page 82, Pat Roberts, letter, December 3, 1992.

Page 83, Roger Peugh, letter, February 9, 1993.

Page 84, Karen, letter, December 4, 1992.

Page 90, Jerry Bridges, **Trusting God**, Colorado Springs, Colorado, NavPress Publishing Group, 1993, page 125. I acknowledge my indebtedness to Mr. Bridges for his summary of the issues presented in this chapter.

Page 90, Bridges, ibid, pages 127–128.

Chapter Nine

Page 91, Joanne Taylor, comments taped at chapel service, November 18,1992.

Page 95, Dayna, poem, undated.

Page 97, Kendra Shultzman, paper, *Impacting My World*, undated.

Page 100, Bonnie Shultzman, poem, August 17, 1993.